How to Make Tofu at Home

A Kitchen Companion for the Curious Home Cook

by M. Eigh

Revised Edition

What Readers Are Saying

How to Make Tofu at Home

★ ★ ★ ★ ★

"This wonderful informative book covers the history of tofu, how it was originally made, and gives the instructions for making it at home — for Tofu, the byproduct Okara, and Soy Milk. You no longer need to buy prepared tofu; you can make your own, starting with the dried beans. Very informative — and very practical instructions!"

— Alex S. • Amazon Verified Purchase

★ ★ ★ ★ ★

"A very interesting Chinese perspective on traditional tofu making. Great cultural information. You can make a batch of tofu in about an hour, and it's much better tasting than anything you will buy at the store."

— Zootal • Amazon Verified Purchase

★ ★ ★ ★ ☆

"Well written, easy to follow instructions and interesting cultural references throughout that put the various processes in historical context. The narrative is also personable which makes reading enjoyable."

— TheFif, United Kingdom • Amazon Verified Purchase

★ ★ ★ ★ ☆

"*Compared to other books on the same subject, this one gives cultural background. I enjoyed it a lot. It discusses the different methods and gives simple instructions.*"

— Dominique, France • Amazon Verified Purchase

. . .

★★★★☆

"*The book is quite interesting, the recipes easy to understand, and it is a way of knowing what is in what you are eating.*"

— Amazon Customer • Amazon Verified Purchase

. . .

A Little Note Before We Begin

I should mention, before we roll up our sleeves, that the FDA and your state may have specific regulations about homemade tofu—things like where your soybeans come from, what tools you use, and who gets to enjoy the finished product. Some states have a Homemade Food Act or a Cottage Food Operation law that covers this sort of thing. If any of that feels murky, it never hurts to check with someone who knows the legal side of things.

This book is simply about the joy of making your own tofu using everyday kitchen tools. Nothing fancy, nothing complicated—just good old-fashioned home cooking.

Dedication

I dedicate this book to King An Liu (劉安, circa 179–122 BC), a remarkable man who—legend has it—invented tofu more than two thousand years ago. What a gift he left us.

I would also like to express my heartfelt thanks to Ms. Daixi for her patient editing help, and to every reader who took the time to share feedback on the first edition. Your kind words and thoughtful suggestions made this new edition possible.

What's Inside

A Brief (and Rather Fascinating) History of Tofu

I remember the first time I really thought about where tofu comes from. I was standing in my kitchen, slicing a block of the stuff for a stir-fry, and it hit me—someone, somewhere, a very long time ago, figured out how to turn a humble little bean into this quietly extraordinary food. And honestly? That story turned out to be far more interesting than I ever expected.

Tofu was born in China roughly two thousand years ago. During the golden age of the Tang Dynasty (618–907 AD), it traveled to Japan and Korea along with so many other treasures of Chinese civilization. The Japanese took to it immediately, and it became a cornerstone of their cuisine. But tofu never lost its place at the Chinese table, either. It spread across every corner of East Asia and, eventually, across the whole world.

Think about it: without tofu, it would have been nearly impossible for Buddhism and its vegetarian traditions to take root and flourish across Asia. In those agrarian civilizations where dairy was practically nonexistent, tofu became *the* source of protein and calcium for millions of people. It still is, for many.

At its heart, tofu is beautifully simple. You coagulate soy milk, press the curds into soft blocks, and there you have it—bean curd. The protein comes from the soybean itself. The calcium? That comes from the original coagulant: gypsum, also known as calcium sulfate. Modern commercial tofu made with calcium chloride is calcium-rich too. And if the maker uses magnesium chloride (called *nigari* in Japan), the tofu picks up a lovely dose of magnesium instead.

The Legend of King An Liu

The Chinese credit a man named An Liu (179–122 BC) with inventing tofu. He was, by all accounts, an extraordinary person—a philosopher, an author, an inventor. While the other royals busied themselves with palace intrigues, An Liu preferred the company of books and the thrill of discovery. He's credited with all sorts of remarkable things, including an early version of the zoetrope and something described as a "flying egg"—an eggshell inflated with steam that floated up into the air—which may have been one of the earliest hot air balloons.

But the tofu story is my favorite, because it starts with love.

Legend has it that An Liu's mother was growing old and frail, and could no longer chew her beloved soybeans. So her devoted son had the beans soaked and ground into a smooth milk, which she could sip easily. Boiled soymilk—still a breakfast staple across China to this day—kept her nourished and content.

Now, An Liu was the curious type. One day (and I imagine he was just puttering around in his alchemy workshop the way I putter around in my kitchen), he dropped a small piece of gypsum rock into a pot of his mother's boiling soymilk. The milk curdled into soft, trembling clumps.

And just like that, tofu was born.

I love that story. The best discoveries often come from someone who simply likes to throw things together and see what happens. I can relate to that—it's basically my approach to weeknight dinners.

Meet Okara: Tofu's Unsung Sibling

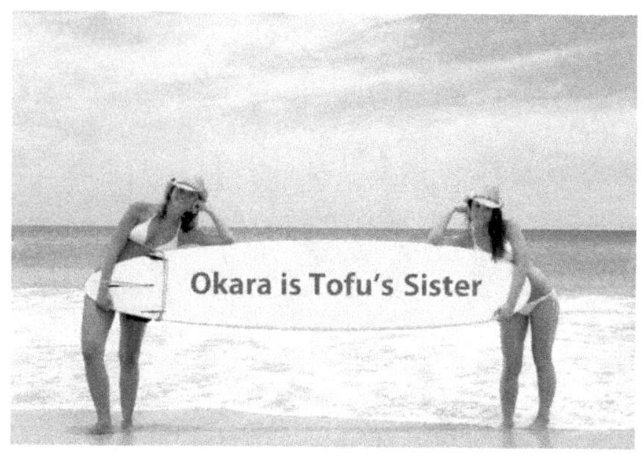

Okara and tofu — two foods born from the same soybean.

First things first: no, I did not misspell "okra." Okara is okara, and it has nothing to do with that lovely green vegetable. (Though I do love okra too, especially fried.)

Okara is the Japanese word (おから) for the soy pulp that's left behind when you strain soymilk out of ground soybeans. The Chinese call it *douzha* (豆渣), and in Korean it's *biji* (비지). I'll stick with "okara" throughout this book, because it rolls off the tongue so nicely.

Here's the thing about okara that fascinates me: every time someone makes tofu, okara is born as a byproduct. They're siblings, really—

two children of the same soybean. The filtered soymilk becomes tofu, and the filtered-out fiber becomes okara. But while tofu has always been treated as a delicacy, poor okara has been looked down on as mere animal feed, or at best, a "filler" for the poor.

Which is such a shame, because nutritionally, okara is a quiet little powerhouse.

The Numbers Tell a Story

Let me share some numbers that might surprise you. Per 100 grams, okara contains about 11.5 grams of dietary fiber—that's three to four times more fiber than broccoli or Brussels sprouts. It delivers protein, carbohydrates, and a nice range of minerals, all for a mere 77 calories. Seventy-seven! For the same serving size, firm tofu delivers about 146 calories but only 0.6 grams of fiber.

Nutrition Facts: Okara (per 100g)

Calories	77
Total Fat	1.7g
Cholesterol	0mg
Sodium	9mg
Total Carbohydrate	13g
Dietary Fiber	11.5g

Protein	3.2g
Calcium	8% DV
Iron	7% DV

Nutrition Facts: Firm Tofu (per 100g)

Calories	146
Total Fat	10g
Cholesterol	0mg
Sodium	2mg
Total Carbohydrate	4.4g
Dietary Fiber	0.6g
Protein	13g
Calcium	34% DV
Iron	15% DV

The dietary fiber in okara is cellulose—the insoluble kind that helps keep your digestive system running smoothly. It aids the intestinal tract, helps with regularity, and may contribute to overall colorectal health. On top of that, okara retains a good proportion of the soybean's calcium and roughly 40% of its protein. The carbohydrates in okara include oligosaccharides and polysaccharides, which are naturally prebiotic—they feed the friendly bacteria in your gut.

So here's what I find delightfully ironic: the very thing that made okara the "poor person's food"—its high fiber and low calories—is exactly what makes it a dream for anyone watching their weight or trying to eat healthier. It fills you up, it's packed with nutrition, and it's practically free because tofu manufacturers are often happy to give it away.

But I'm getting ahead of myself. Let's make some tofu first, and the okara will take care of itself.

Let's Make Tofu!

This is the part I get genuinely excited about. Making tofu at home sounds like it should be complicated, but I promise you, it's really not. If you can make oatmeal, you can make tofu. (Well, maybe tofu requires a tiny bit more patience than oatmeal. But only a tiny bit.)

When I was growing up in China, my family used to make tofu every Sunday. The whole family pitched in—my mother soaked the soybeans, my sisters fed them into the stone grinder with just the right amount of water, my brothers and I cranked the grinder by hand, and my father did the all-important job of dropping the coagulant into the boiling wok at precisely the right moment. Those Sunday mornings are some of my fondest memories. The kitchen smelled incredible, everyone was laughing, and by lunchtime we had the freshest tofu you can imagine.

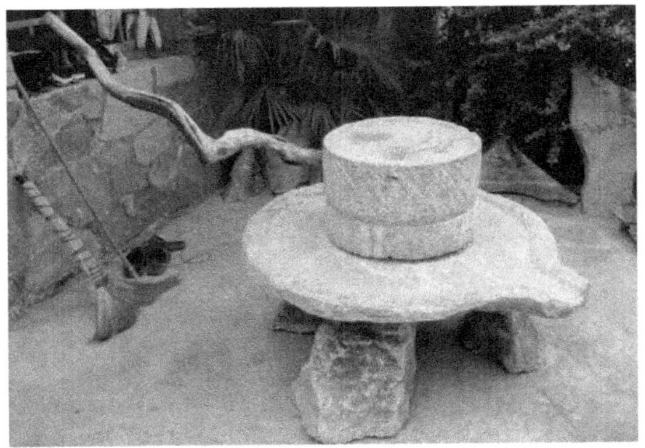

An ancient stone soy grinder — the traditional tool now replaced by the household blender.

Back then, houses in China were built around courtyards, and there were always communal stone grinders sitting in the open atrium. Families took turns using and cleaning the grinders, and every year the community pooled money to hire a mason to re-groove the grinding surfaces. You can only see those old grinders in museums now, or in some very remote countryside villages. But the tofu—thankfully—lives on.

Today, of course, you don't need a stone grinder. A regular kitchen blender does the job perfectly. Here's what you'll need to get started:

What You'll Need

• A blender (a regular household blender works wonderfully—please use a blender, not a juicer, as a juicer gives poor yields and might even get damaged)

• Two deep pots

• A colander

• A few pieces of cheesecloth (or a clean cotton cloth)

• Dried soybeans (readily available at any supermarket)

• A coagulant (I'll explain your options in a moment)

• A heavy flat object for pressing (a plate with a can on top works fine)

That's it. No special equipment, no hard-to-find gadgets. Just simple kitchen things you probably already have.

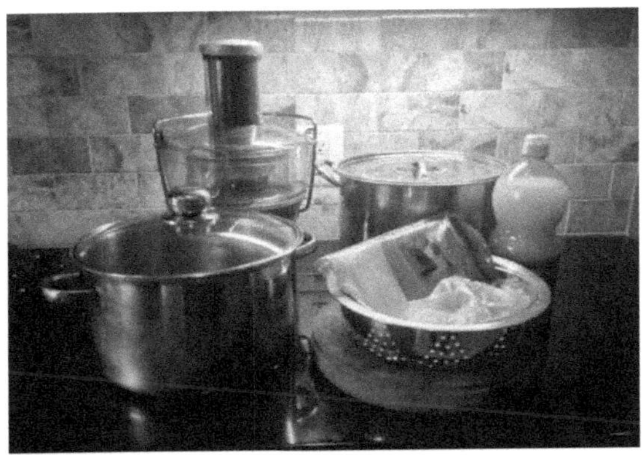

Home setup: two pots, blender, cheesecloth, and coagulant. Everything you need.

Step 1: Soak and Blend

We eat a lot of tofu in my house, so for this walk-through I started with three cups of dried soybeans. If you're just dipping your toes in, one and a half to two cups is plenty for a first batch.

I like to buy organic, non-GMO soybeans when I can find them. My thinking is, if I'm already going to the trouble of making my own tofu, I might as well start with the best beans I can get. But honestly? Regular dried soybeans from any grocery store will work just fine. Use what you have and don't let perfect be the enemy of good tofu.

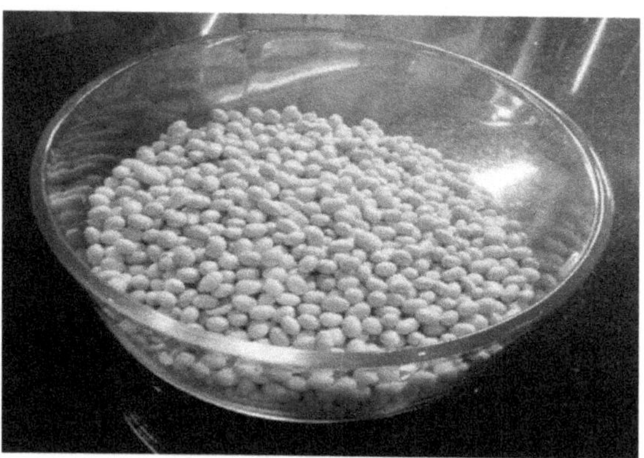

Dried soybeans before soaking.

Soaking: Place your dried beans in a large bowl—and I do mean large, because they'll expand to three or four times their original size overnight. Cover them generously with cool water and pop the bowl in the fridge. Let them soak for at least eight hours, or just overnight.

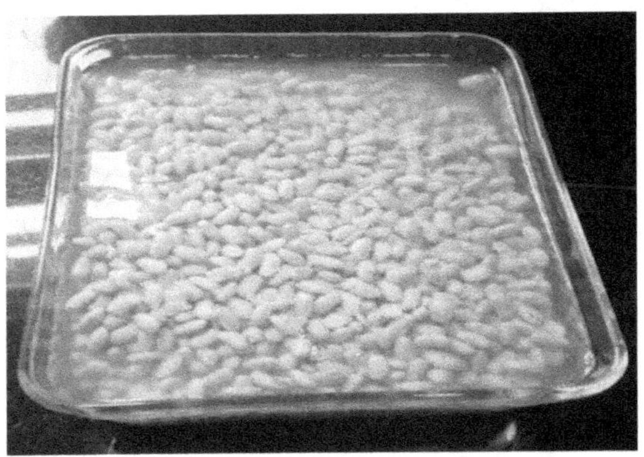

Soaked and ready — soybeans expand nearly four times in volume.

A little tip: the soaking time does depend on temperature. In cold water (around 10–15°C), plan for 12 to 16 hours. In warmer water (15–20°C), 8 to 10 hours should do it. The beans should feel plump and smooth when they're ready—split one open and the inside should be uniformly colored with no dry, opaque center.

Blending: Divide your soaked beans into two or three batches (my blender does best with manageable portions). For each batch, add roughly an equal amount of water—about a 1:1 ratio of soaked beans to water. You'll notice some loose bean skins floating around in your soaking water. Leave them in! They're full of good antioxidants.

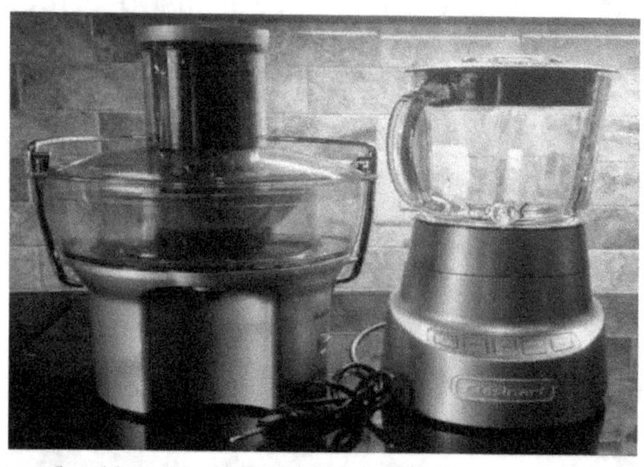

A standard household blender is perfectly adequate for the job.

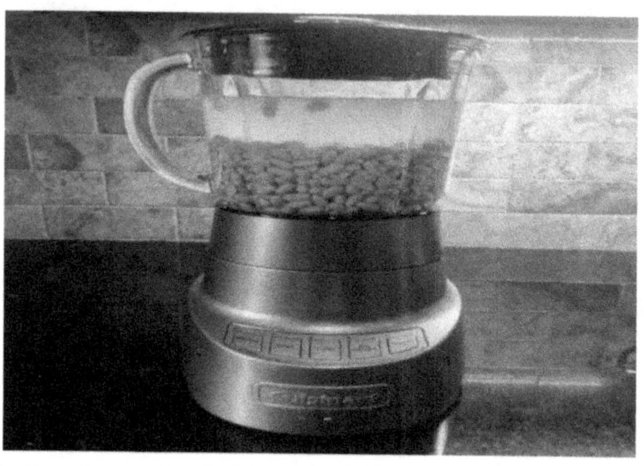

Soaked soybeans loaded into the blender with water, ready to pulp.

Blend each batch until you have a smooth, creamy pulp. It should look like a thick, pale smoothie. If your blender struggles, add a splash more water. The goal is a uniformly smooth texture with no visible bean chunks—the finer the grind, the more soymilk you'll extract.

Step 2: From Soy Pulp to Silky Soymilk (and Okara!)

Now comes the part that feels a little like magic. You're going to separate the soymilk from the okara, and suddenly you'll have two wonderful ingredients instead of one.

Straining: Line your colander with a double layer of cheesecloth and set it over one of your deep pots. Pour the blended soy pulp into the colander, a batch at a time.

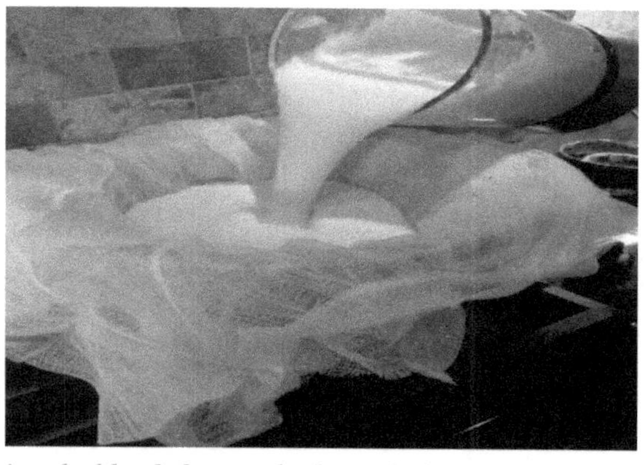

Pouring the blended soy pulp through cheesecloth into the pot.

Squeezing: This is where you earn your tofu. Gather the cheesecloth into a bundle and squeeze, wring, and press out as much soymilk as you possibly can. Really get in there—the more milk you extract, the more tofu you'll end up with. My mother always said you're not done squeezing until your arms are tired. She wasn't wrong.

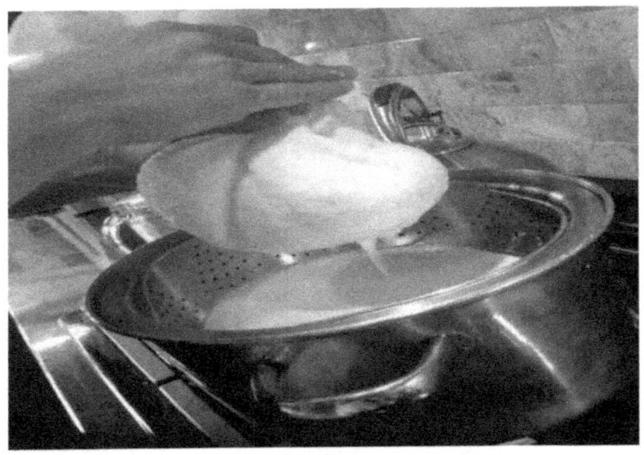

Squeezing the cheesecloth firmly — extract every drop of soymilk.

The milky white liquid streaming into your pot? That's your soymilk—liquid gold, as far as I'm concerned. And the fibrous pulp left in the cheesecloth? That's your okara. Set it aside (I'll tell you what to do with it later—don't you dare throw it away!).

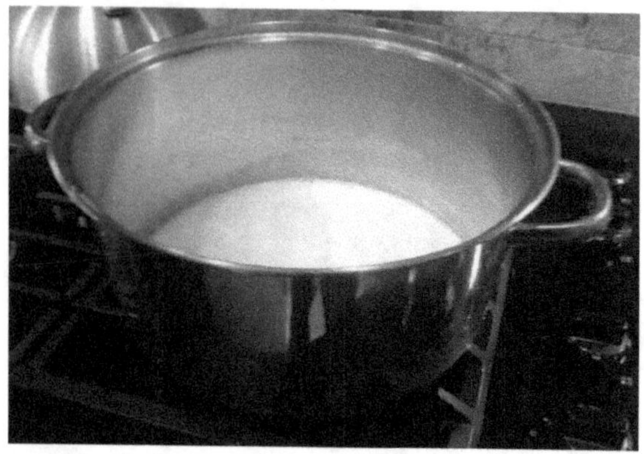

Fresh soymilk in the pot — thin, raw, and ready to simmer.

A note on method: What I've just described is the traditional Chinese method of *cold filtering*—you strain the raw, uncooked pulp. Many online tutorials will tell you to boil the pulp first, and then filter. Both methods work, but I prefer the traditional cold-filtering approach for three reasons:

First, the soymilk curdles into tofu more reliably when the okara has been filtered out while cold. *Second*, cold-separated okara tastes noticeably better—less mushy, more pleasant. And *third*, cold-filtered okara freezes beautifully in zip-top bags, staying fresh for months.

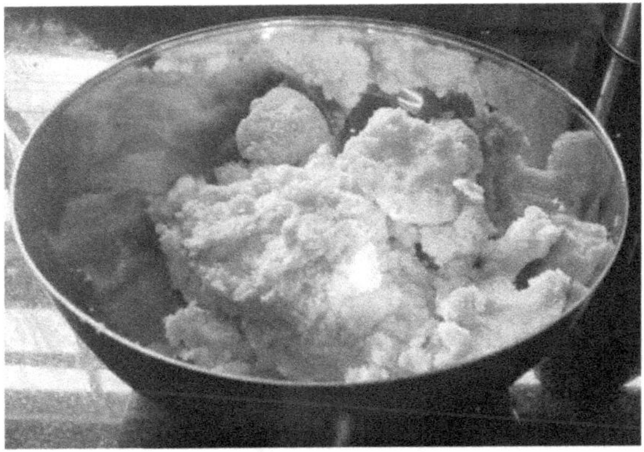

Fresh okara — the fiber-rich pulp remaining after straining.

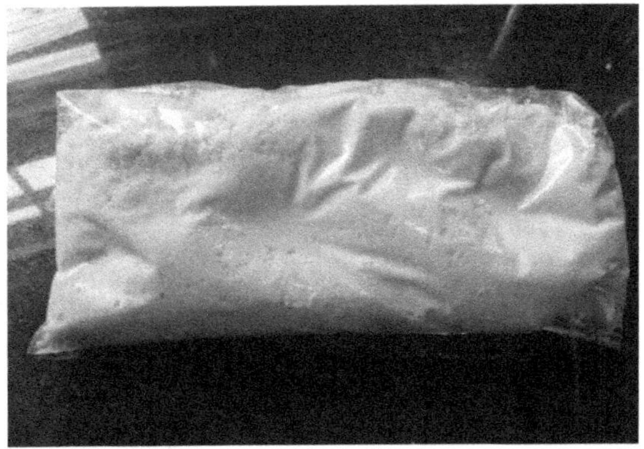

Surplus okara zip-bagged and ready for the freezer. Keeps well for months.

Adjusting the milk: The soymilk straight from the blender will be quite thick. For tofu-making, a ratio of about 1 part soaked soybeans to 2–3 parts total water works well. If your milk seems very thick, stir in an additional cup or two of water until it has the consistency of whole cow's milk. Don't thin it too much, though—you need enough protein in there for the curds to form properly.

If you made extra, this is a lovely time to ladle out a bowl or two of soymilk to enjoy later. Boiled soymilk with a pinch of sugar is a traditional Chinese breakfast that I still crave. (Though it's wonderful plain, too, or with a drizzle of honey.)

Step 3: The Magic of Curdling

This is the moment. This is where soymilk becomes tofu. I still find it thrilling, every single time.

Boil the soymilk: Pour your soymilk into a clean, deep pot and bring it to a boil over medium-high heat. A boil is important—it kills any bacteria in the raw milk and also deactivates something called trypsin inhibitor, which can upset your stomach if the milk isn't heated properly. You should let the soymilk simmer for a good 10–15 minutes to be safe.

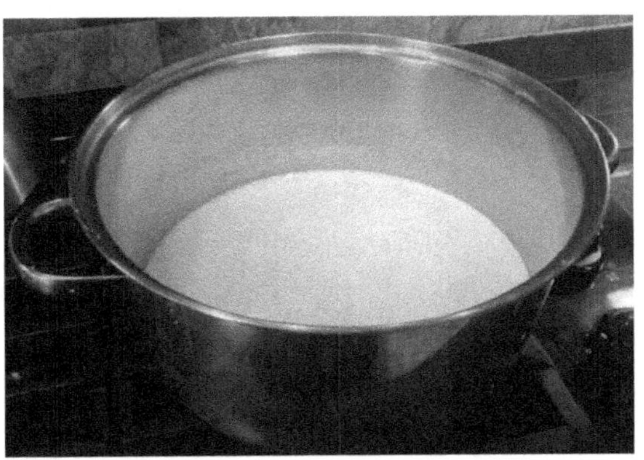

Soymilk just coming to a boil — watch for the first rolling bubbles.

Keep an eye on it, though! Soymilk loves to foam up and boil over at the most inconvenient moment. Stir gently and watch it like you'd watch a pot of regular milk. A little foam on top is perfectly normal. If it threatens to overflow, just lower the heat for a moment.

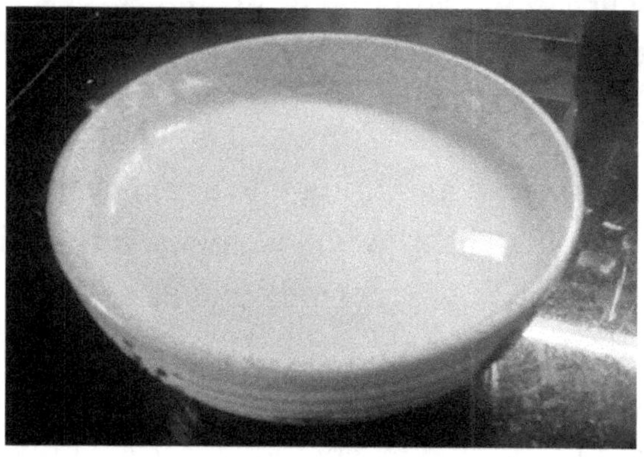

Scoop out drinking soymilk now, before adding any coagulant.

Prepare your coagulant: While the soymilk heats, get your coagulant ready. I'll discuss coagulant options in detail in the next section, but here's the quick version: if you're using lemon juice or vinegar, warm about two-thirds of a cup in a separate pot. If you're using a salt coagulant like gypsum or nigari, dissolve the appropriate amount in a cup of warm water.

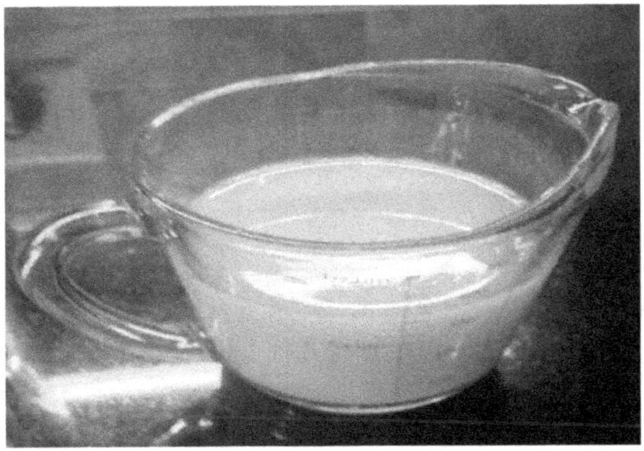

Lemon juice measured and warmed — the most accessible beginner coagulant.

The pour: Here's a technique my father taught me, passed down through our family: the traditional Chinese "poured, not stirred" method. Once your soymilk is at a gentle boil, pour it from as high as you can comfortably manage into the pot containing your coagulant. Pour forcefully and try to hit every part of the pot's bottom. This technique ensures thorough, even mixing without the need for stirring.

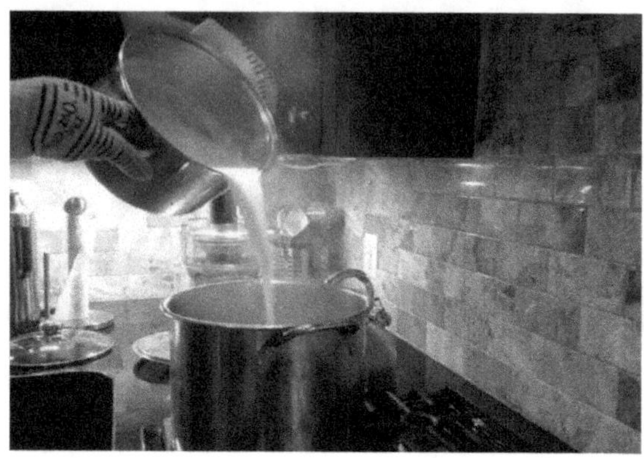

The high pour — raise the pot as high as you can. The turbulent mixing does the work.

The wait: After the pour, *do not stir*. I know it's tempting. Put the lid on and walk away for 15 to 20 minutes. You can reheat the pot gently to keep it near-boiling temperature, but don't bring it to a full boil, and please don't stir. Both boiling and stirring disrupt the delicate curdling process and can leave you with a grainy, uneven texture.

After about 15 minutes, lift the lid and take a peek. If everything went well, you should see soft, white curds floating in a clear, pale-yellow liquid (that's the whey). If the liquid is still milky or cloudy, the coagulation isn't complete—you may need a touch more coagulant or a few more minutes of resting time.

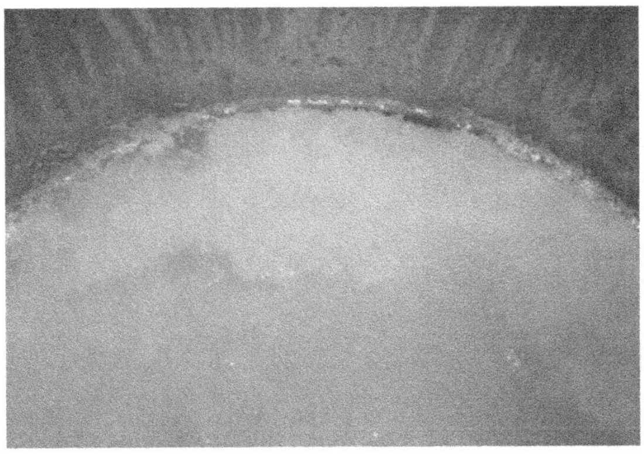

Curds forming in the whey — 15 minutes after the pour. Do not stir.

Congratulations!—you've just made silken tofu. Technically, these trembling curds are already edible. If you're making miso soup, just scoop some directly into the broth. It's heavenly.

Pressing into firm tofu: For most cooking, though, you'll want something firmer. Line your colander with cheesecloth, gently ladle or pour the curds in, and fold the cheesecloth over the top. Place a flat plate on top, and then add weight—a heavy can, a pot of water, even a clean brick. The idea is gentle, steady pressure to squeeze out the whey.

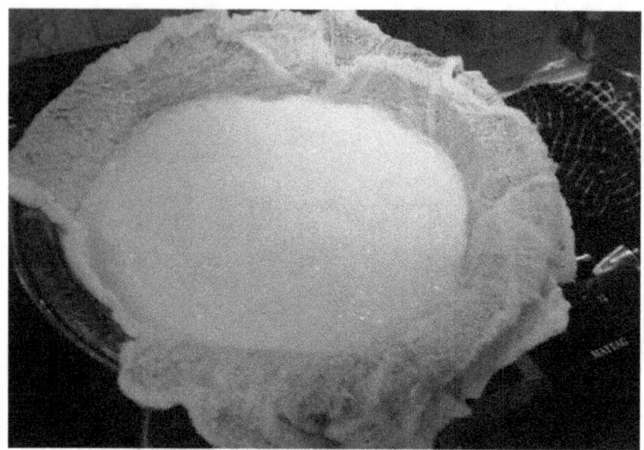

Ladling the curds into the cheesecloth-lined colander.

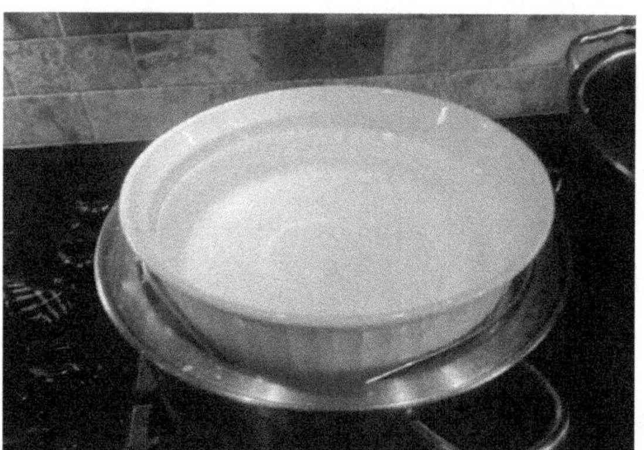

A heavy bowl weighted on top presses the curds into a firm block.

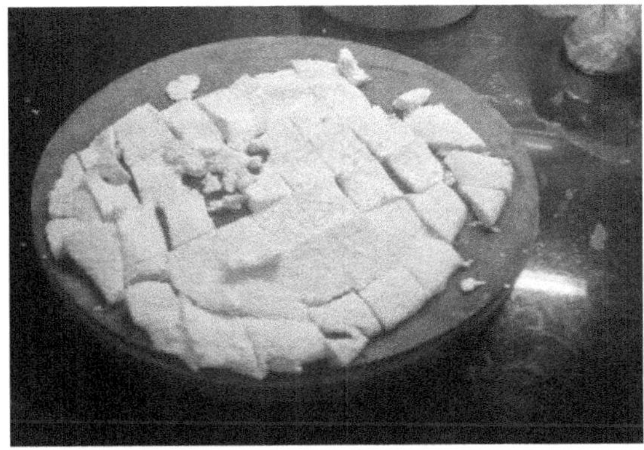

Apply steady, even pressure for 15–30 minutes.

Leave it for 15 to 20 minutes for soft tofu, or 30 minutes to an hour for something firmer. You'll get a feel for it after your first batch.

Once pressed, gently unwrap your tofu and place it in a bowl of cold water for about 30 minutes. This firms up the texture a bit more and, if you used an acid coagulant, helps wash away any lingering tang or bitterness.

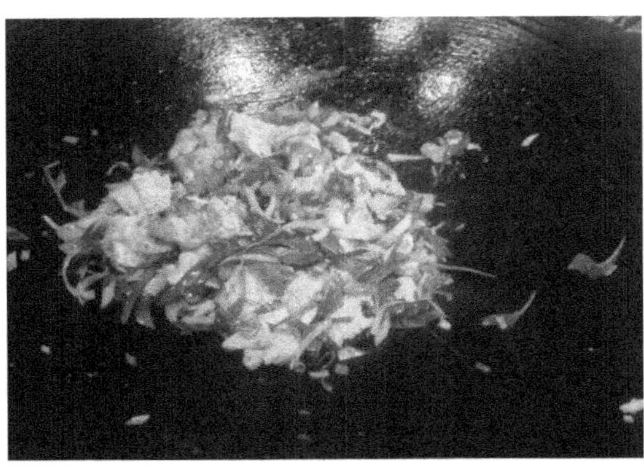

And there it is. Your very own block of fresh, homemade tofu. I promise you, the first time you slice into it and realize *you made this*, it feels like a small miracle.

A Quick Word About Coagulants

This is the part that confused me the most when I first started, so I want to take a moment to walk you through your options. The coagulant you choose really does make a difference in the flavor, texture, and overall quality of your tofu.

Salt Coagulants (My Recommendation)

Gypsum (Calcium Sulfate): This is the traditional Chinese coagulant—the very same substance King An Liu is said to have used over two thousand years ago. It reacts gently with soymilk, producing curds with wonderful water-holding capacity and a soft, smooth texture. The resulting tofu has a mild, clean taste. Gypsum is easy to use and very forgiving, which makes it lovely for beginners. It also boosts the calcium content of your tofu beautifully. You can find food-grade calcium sulfate online or at specialty stores.

Nigari (Magnesium Chloride): This is the traditional Japanese coagulant—salt crystals derived from seawater. Nigari gives tofu a subtly sweet, almost delicate flavor that many people consider the gold standard. It does work faster and more aggressively than gypsum, so it requires a bit more attention when adding it. The tofu may be slightly less smooth than gypsum tofu, but the flavor is exquisite. You can often find nigari at health food stores or Asian grocery shops. When buying, check the label—some products are diluted and you may need to adjust the amount.

Acid Coagulants

Lemon juice, vinegar, or other acids: These work in a pinch and they're certainly convenient—everyone has a lemon or a bottle of vinegar on hand. However, I should be upfront: acid coagulants do leave a noticeable tangy flavor in the finished tofu, and the texture tends to be slightly crumbly compared to what you get with salt coagulants. If you're brand new to tofu-making and just want to try the process once to see how it works, lemon juice is perfectly fine. But if you plan to make tofu regularly, I'd really encourage you to invest in some gypsum or nigari. The difference is remarkable.

GDL (Glucono-delta-lactone): This is what commercial manufacturers use for silken tofu. It produces a very smooth, uniform curd, but the tofu can have a slightly sour taste, especially in firmer versions. GDL is available online if you want to experiment.

How Much Coagulant?

As a general guide for soymilk made from about 3 cups of dried soybeans:

• **Gypsum:** 2–3 teaspoons, dissolved in 1 cup of warm water

• **Nigari:** about 1–2 teaspoons (start with less—you can always add more)

• **Lemon juice or vinegar:** about ⅔ cup

The right amount depends on how concentrated your soymilk is. Here's a lovely trick from the pros: watch the whey. When you've added enough coagulant, the liquid above the curds will turn clear and slightly yellowish. If it's still cloudy, you need a bit more. If the curds look chunky and the whey is very clear, you may have slightly overdone it—

but don't worry, the tofu will still be perfectly good.

Temperature matters too. You want the soymilk to be around 75–85°C (roughly 165–185°F) when you add the coagulant. Too hot and the reaction happens too fast, giving you a harder, drier tofu. Too cool and the curds won't form properly. If you have a kitchen thermometer, this is a nice time to use it—but after a batch or two, you'll develop an instinct for it.

Cooking with Your Fresh Tofu

The very first thing I do with a fresh batch of homemade tofu is the simplest thing imaginable: I stir-fry it with leeks. Just a splash of oil in a hot wok, some sliced leeks, cubes of your fresh tofu, a drizzle of soy sauce, and dinner is ready in five minutes. The tofu is so flavorful on its own that it barely needs anything.

But of course, fresh tofu is wonderfully versatile. What follows is a collection of my family's favorites, along with ideas I've gathered from friends, neighbors, and fellow tofu enthusiasts over the years. Think of this as a little window-shopping tour through the world of tofu cooking—browse at your leisure, dog-ear the ones that catch your eye, and come back to them whenever the mood strikes.

Family Favorites

Mapo Tofu: The classic Sichuan dish—soft tofu in a fiery, numbing sauce with ground pork. If you've never had it, you're in for a treat. If you have, imagine how much better it tastes with tofu you made yourself. The secret is in the *doubanjiang* (fermented chili bean paste)—just a couple of tablespoons transforms everything. Swirl in some Sichuan peppercorns at the end for that tingly, mouth-numbing magic that makes this dish legendary.

Pan-Fried Tofu with Dipping Sauce: Slice your tofu into thick planks, pat them dry, and pan-fry in a bit of oil until golden on both sides. Serve with a dipping sauce of soy sauce, rice vinegar, sesame oil, and a pinch of chili flakes. This is my go-to lazy dinner and it never disappoints. A friend in Chengdu taught me to dust the slices with a pinch of Chinese five-spice powder before frying—the aroma alone will bring people running to the kitchen.

Miso Soup: Simply scoop your silken curds (before pressing!) into a bowl of warm miso broth with some wakame seaweed and thinly sliced scallions. This is comfort in a bowl. I learned this from my Japanese neighbor, Mrs. Tanaka, who insists that the miso should never actually boil—you stir it in at the very end, off the heat, to keep those lovely live cultures intact.

Sweet and Sour Tofu: Cubed firm tofu, lightly coated in cornstarch and fried until crisp, then tossed in a tangy sweet-and-sour sauce with bell peppers and pineapple. A crowd-pleaser, every time. The trick is getting those cubes really crispy before the sauce goes on—give them space in the pan so they fry rather than steam.

Tofu and Bok Choy Soup: A gentle, nourishing soup that's perfect for chilly evenings. The tofu adds protein and the bok choy brings a lovely fresh crunch. I like to drop in a few slices of fresh ginger and a splash of white pepper—it warms you right through.

Scrambled Tofu: Crumble firm tofu into a pan with a little turmeric, nutritional yeast, and your favorite vegetables. It's a beautiful plant-based breakfast. My daughter adds black salt (*kala namak*) for an eggy flavor that fools everyone at the table.

More Ideas to Explore

Once you've made tofu a few times and have a steady supply in your fridge, you'll start seeing possibilities everywhere. Here are more dishes worth trying—some traditional, some creative, all delicious.

Kung Pao Tofu: If you love the classic chicken version, you'll adore this. Cube your firm tofu, fry until the edges are crispy, then toss with roasted peanuts, diced celery, and a sticky-savory sauce of soy sauce, rice vinegar, a touch of sugar, and dried red chilies. The peanuts add crunch, the chilies add heat, and the tofu soaks up every bit of that gorgeous sauce. It comes together in about fifteen minutes—weeknight perfection.

Crispy Sesame Tofu: Press your firm tofu well, cut into bite-sized rectangles, and coat lightly in cornstarch. Pan-fry until all sides are golden and crunchy. Then toss in a glaze of soy sauce, maple syrup, rice vinegar, sesame oil, and a generous sprinkling of sesame seeds. The contrast between the crispy exterior and the creamy interior is absolutely addictive. My kids eat these faster than I can make them.

Steamed Tofu with Chili Sauce: This is the gentlest, most elegant way to enjoy fresh tofu. Simply slice your softest tofu into a shallow dish, steam for five minutes, then drizzle with a sauce of soy sauce, chili oil, minced garlic, and a whisper of sugar. Scatter some chopped scallions and cilantro on top. It's the kind of dish that really lets the flavor of your homemade tofu shine—clean, delicate, and honest.

Pan-Fried Tofu with Black Bean Sauce: Fermented black beans (*douchi*) are one of China's great secret weapons. Pan-fry your tofu slices until golden, set them aside, then quickly stir-fry garlic, ginger, and a tablespoon of fermented black beans in the same pan. Add a splash of soy sauce and a little water to make a sauce, return the tofu, and let everything mingle for a minute. The deep, umami richness of those fermented beans paired with fresh homemade tofu is something special.

Tofu Skin Rolls (Yuba):* Here's a bonus if you're patient: while boiling your soymilk, you'll notice a thin skin forming on the surface. That's yuba—tofu skin—and it's considered a delicacy. Carefully lift it off with chopsticks, let it cool, and roll it up with julienned vegetables and a drizzle of sesame oil. My grandmother used to say the tofu skin belonged to whoever was watching the pot. Naturally, I always volunteered.

Agedashi Tofu: A beloved Japanese preparation. Coat cubes of soft tofu in potato starch (or cornstarch) and deep-fry until the outside is delicately crisp. Serve in a warm pool of dashi broth seasoned with soy sauce and mirin, topped with grated daikon, sliced scallions, and a pinch of bonito flakes. The tofu puffs up slightly in the fryer, and when you bite through that thin, crispy shell into the silky center—pure bliss.

Stuffed Tofu (Niang Doufu):* A Hakka classic. Cut firm tofu blocks in half, scoop out a small well in each piece, and stuff with a mixture of minced pork, shrimp, and water chestnuts seasoned with soy sauce and sesame oil. Pan-fry stuffed-side down until golden, then braise in a light broth. Every region has its own version—some stuff with fish paste, some with mushrooms. It's the kind of dish that looks impressive but is really quite simple once you get the hang of it.

Tofu Pudding (Douhua):* If you stop the tofu-making process right after adding the coagulant—before pressing—you get the silkiest, most tender curd imaginable. In southern China, we serve it warm with a ginger syrup. In Sichuan, they go savory with chili oil, soy sauce, crushed peanuts, and pickled vegetables. Either way, it's essentially the "first fruits" of your tofu-making, and it's divine. I always scoop out a small bowl of douhua for myself before I press the rest into blocks. Cook's privilege.

*Cold Tofu Salad (Hiyayakko):** Another Japanese gem that requires almost no cooking at all. Chill a block of your freshest, softest tofu, place it on a pretty plate, and top with grated fresh ginger, sliced scallions, bonito flakes, and a drizzle of soy sauce. That's it. The Japanese have a wonderful instinct for letting good ingredients speak for themselves, and this dish is the purest expression of that philosophy. On a hot summer evening, there's nothing better.

Minced Pork and Tofu Fritters: These are wonderful as appetizers or tucked into lunch boxes. Crumble your tofu and mix with minced pork, finely chopped scallions, a beaten egg, a spoonful of cornstarch, and seasonings of your choice (I like a touch of five-spice). Shape into small patties or balls and pan-fry or deep-fry until golden. They're crispy outside, tender inside, and disappear alarmingly fast at parties.

The wonderful thing about homemade tofu is that it absorbs flavors even better than store-bought, because it's fresher and hasn't been sitting in preservative-laden water for days. Season it boldly and it will reward you. And don't be afraid to experiment—some of my best tofu dishes came from happy accidents and whatever happened to be in the fridge that evening.

Okara: The Miracle You Almost Threw Away

Remember that soft, damp pulp left in your cheesecloth after straining? Please tell me you didn't toss it. Because okara, my friend, is a treasure.

If you've been buying tofu at the store, you've never even met okara. It simply doesn't exist in the retail world—tofu manufacturers either sell it cheaply as animal feed or throw it away. Which is a terrible waste, because okara is one of the most nutritious, most versatile, and most underappreciated foods I know.

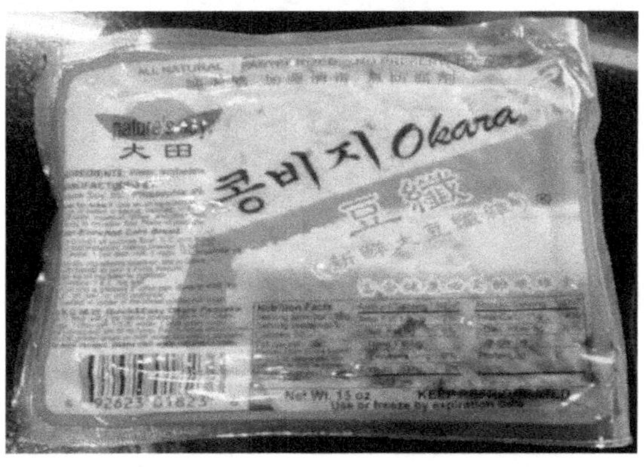

Packaged okara from an Asian supermarket — look in the tofu section.

I've already shared the nutrition numbers, so you know it's loaded with fiber (11.5 grams per

100g!), has plenty of protein and minerals, and carries barely any calories. It fills you up, it keeps your digestive system happy, and it's essentially free when you make your own tofu. What's not to love?

Here are a few of my favorite things to do with fresh okara:

Stir-fried okara: Sauté it with chopped shiitake mushrooms, carrots, and a drizzle of sesame oil. Add a splash of soy sauce and mirin. This is a traditional Japanese dish called *unohana* and it's absolutely delicious—earthy, savory, and satisfying.

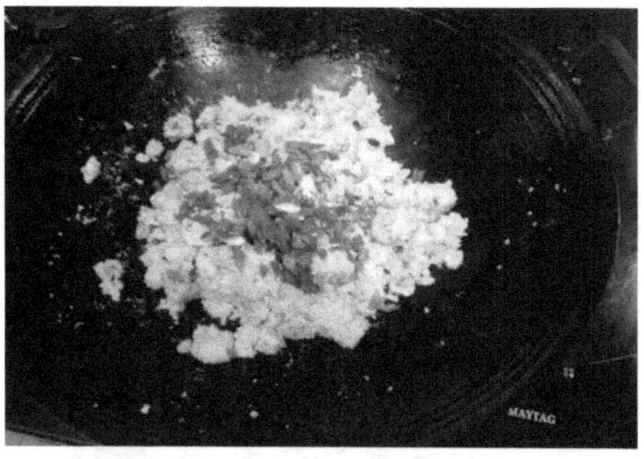

Okara stir-frying in a wok with scallions.

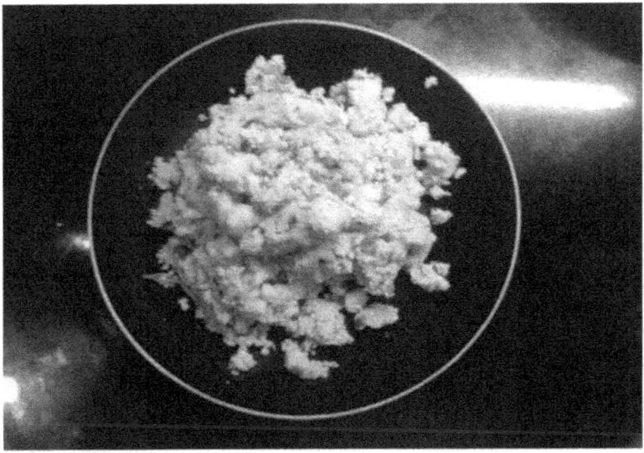

The finished dish — simple, savory, and remarkably filling.

Okara patties: Mix okara with breadcrumbs, chopped scallions, a beaten egg, and whatever seasonings you like. Shape into patties and pan-fry until golden. These are wonderful with a dipping sauce or tucked into a sandwich.

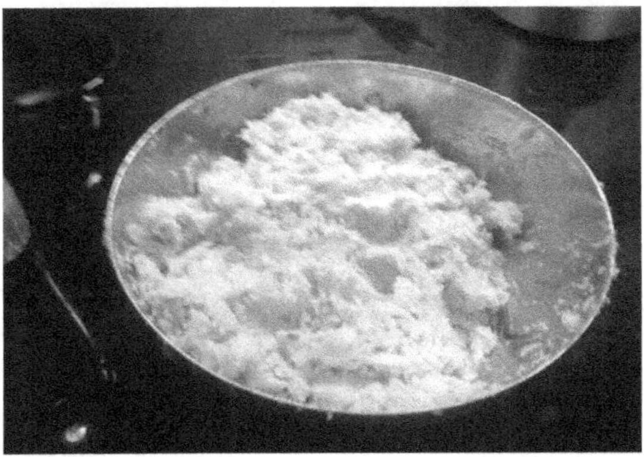

Okara patty mixture — the binder holds together beautifully.

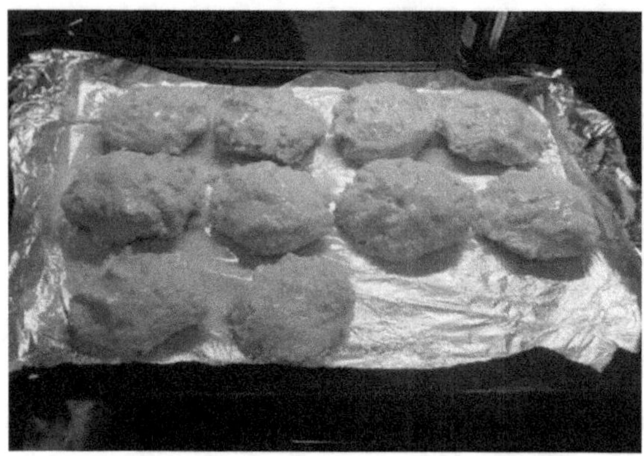

Patties shaped and ready for the oven.

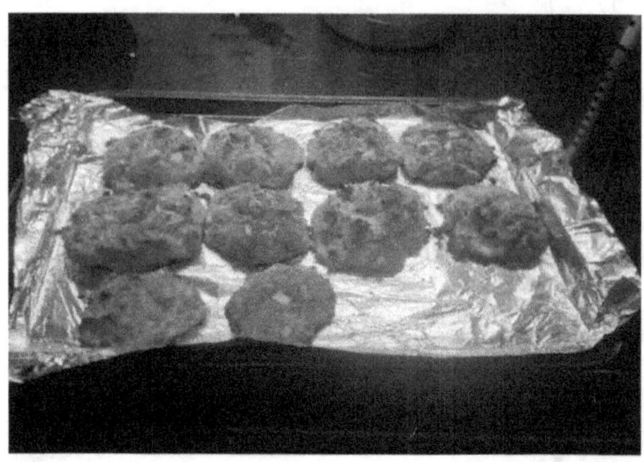

Golden and crisped — serve with lemon wedges and your choice of sauce.

In baking: You can substitute okara for part of the flour in muffins, quick breads, and pancakes. It adds moisture, fiber, and a subtle nuttiness. Start by replacing about a quarter of the flour and adjust from there.

Smoothie booster: A spoonful of okara blended into your morning smoothie adds fiber and protein without changing the flavor much.

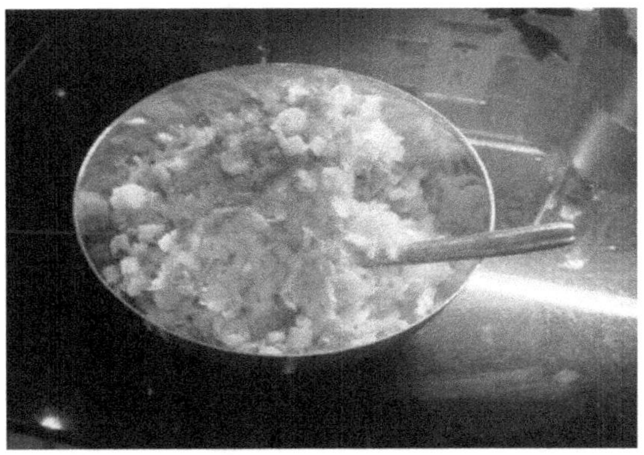

Okara salad — a protein-rich, high-fiber meal in minutes.

Storage tip: Fresh okara keeps in the fridge for two or three days. If you've made more than you can use right away (and you probably will), portion it into zip-top bags, flatten them out, and freeze. It keeps beautifully for months. When you're ready to use it, just thaw in the fridge overnight.

If you're interested in diving deeper into the remarkable health benefits and culinary possibilities of okara, I wrote a companion book called *Lose Weight with Okara: A Miracle Food,* which is part dietary guide and

part culinary adventure. It's available on
Amazon.

Frequently Asked Questions

Over the years, readers have asked me all sorts of wonderful questions. Here are the ones that come up most often:

Can I use store-bought soymilk to make tofu?

You can try, but I wouldn't recommend it for your best batch. Most commercial soymilk is too diluted and contains additives (sweeteners, flavors, stabilizers) that interfere with the curdling process. If you want to experiment, look for unsweetened soymilk with the shortest ingredient list you can find, and use extra coagulant. But really, making your own soymilk from whole beans is so easy and the results are so much better.

My tofu has a spread-like texture, more like cream cheese. What went wrong?

This usually means either not enough coagulant, or the soymilk wasn't hot enough when the coagulant was added. Try using a bit more coagulant next time, and make sure your milk is around 75–85°C. Also, let the curds rest a full 15–20 minutes before pressing.

What kind of water should I use?

Tofu is about 80% water, so water quality genuinely matters. Soft water (with less calcium and magnesium) tends to produce better-tasting tofu. If your tap water is very hard, consider using filtered water. If you have naturally soft well water or spring water, you're in luck—that's ideal.

My tofu tastes bitter or sour. How do I fix that?

Bitterness usually comes from the coagulant—especially if you used a bit too much nigari or Epsom salt. Sourness comes from acid coagulants like lemon juice or vinegar. In either case, soaking the finished tofu in cold water for 30 minutes to an hour will help wash away the off-flavors. For future batches, switch to gypsum (calcium sulfate) for the cleanest, mildest taste.

I burned the soymilk while heating it. Help!

Oh, I've been there. Soymilk scorches easily if you're not stirring regularly. When you bring the milk to a boil, use medium heat and stir gently and frequently—vertical, horizontal, and diagonal strokes, touching the bottom of the pot. A heavy-bottomed pot helps too. If you do burn it, carefully pour the milk into a new pot, leaving the scorched layer behind. The tofu may have a slight off-taste, but it's usually still fine.

Can I make tofu without any special coagulant?

In a pinch, yes—lemon juice or white vinegar from your pantry will work. But for truly good tofu, I'd encourage you to order some food-grade calcium sulfate (gypsum) or nigari online. They're inexpensive, they last forever, and the difference in quality is remarkable.

How long does homemade tofu keep?

Stored in a container of fresh water in the fridge (change the water daily), homemade tofu keeps for about 3–5 days. But honestly? In my house, it never lasts that long.

What about Epsom salt as a coagulant?

Some people use Epsom salt (magnesium sulfate) and it does work. However, I'm a little cautious about it because the Epsom salt sold in drugstores is typically marketed as a bath soak, not a food product. There's no evidence it's unsafe, but there's also no explicit food-grade certification on most packages. If you want a magnesium-based coagulant, I'd suggest seeking out nigari instead—it's specifically made for tofu and you'll know exactly what you're getting.

A Few Parting Thoughts

If you made it this far, thank you. Truly. Whether you're reading this on a lazy afternoon, or with your sleeves already rolled up and soybeans soaking in the kitchen, I hope this little book has made the world of homemade tofu feel approachable, maybe even exciting.

Making tofu at home isn't just about saving money (though you will—store-bought tofu can cost more per pound than pork chops, and a bag of dried soybeans goes a remarkably long way). It's about connection. Connection to a tradition that stretches back two millennia. Connection to the simple, beautiful chemistry of turning beans into something extraordinary. And maybe, if you're lucky, connection to the people in your kitchen who pitch in to help.

My family doesn't crank a stone grinder anymore. But we still make tofu together. My daughters fight over who gets to squeeze the cheesecloth. My husband still insists on being the one to add the coagulant, just like my father did. And every time I slice into a fresh block of warm, trembling tofu, I think of An Liu and his mother, and I smile.

Go make some tofu. And please, *please* don't throw away the okara.

With warmth and soy-stained hands,

M. Eigh

I'd love to hear about your tofu adventures. You can find me and my other books on Amazon by searching for M. Eigh.

www.ingramcontent.com/pod-product-compliance
Lightning Source LLC
Chambersburg PA
CBHW051010050726

47592CB00007B/2783